JUST FOR TODAY

By Franca J. Navarra

CONTENTS

Title Page	
Dedication	
Acknowledgement	
Preface	1
Day 1	9
Day 2	10
Day 3	11
Day 4	12
Day 5	13
Day 6	15
Day 7	17
Day 8	19
Day 9	20
Day 10	21
Day 11	23
Day 12	25

Day 13	27
Day 14	28
Day 15	29
Day 16	30
Day 17	31
Day 18	32
Day 19	34
Day 20	37
Day 21	38
Day 22	40
Day 23	42
Day 24	43
Day 25	45
Day 26	47
Day 27	49
Day 28	51
Day 29	52
Day 30	53
About The Author	55
SOURCES AND REFERENCES	56

DEDICATION

This book is dedicated to everyone who believes in the power of self love.

ACKNOWLEDGEMENT

I would like to acknowledge and thank all the inspiring and knowledgeable teachers and coaches who I have worked with over the years. Because of you, I have gained the tools, strategies, and wisdom needed to enrich my life on so many levels. It's been a privilege and I am honoured to pass on this book to help others along their journey to a more fulfilling life. May you find love within yourself.

Special thanks to Holly Cambruzzi for editing this book.

My Message to You

Deliberately make yourself the priority, reason and purpose of your existence.

This book is a reminder you all have the power to create a happy and fulfilling life.

I know first hand life can present challenges that can set off a whirlwind of emotions.

I too struggled with love, raising my sons as a single mother, and finding time for myself.

One day it dawned on me, if I wanted to experience happiness, love, and balance, the change had to start from within.

And so, my journey began. I adopted a new

empowered mindset, and transformed myself from a once directionless, anxious, and unhappy woman, to living a more vibrant, joyous, and meaningful life.

Today, I use my experiences to help others gain hope, clarity, and strength, so they too can fall in love with themselves and their lives again.

This guide is a representation of some of the most impactful life strategies and tools which I have applied to enhance my own life, and become the woman I am today.

I am delightfully honoured to share the insights and knowledge needed to guide you to a more meaningful, vibrant, and fulfilling life.

Love

Franca J. Navarra

PREFACE

Just for Today...

30 Day Challenge to Change

You Got this Thing Called Life!

So often most people walk around as if the weight of the world is on their shoulders.

Although it may feel like it at times, one thing is certain, you can change it.

This is not rocket science, real change or growth can only happen if you are willing to adjust your approach and do things differently.

This applies to all areas of your life. In order to get different results, you must take different actions or you will create the same outcome.

You see, change and growth are intertwined like life and time.

As soon as you make the decision to change, growth immediately takes place. Know this, there is great power in your decisions. When you make the decision to change, it comes from a place of clarity. This awareness required you to tune into yourself and re-evaluate all areas of your life. This valuable component is what will start you along a path towards growth, enhancement, and a better life.

This book is designed to help you relax as you embark on your journey to creating a happier, more meaningful and fulfilling life. By making small, yet significant daily changes you can experience more positive emotions, improve your relationships, attract great manifestations, and so much more..., -the benefits are endless.

All you must do right now is decide if you are up for the challenge to change.

Because your willingness to want to make changes, transformations, and improvements, growth will naturally happen.

Just start with where you are right now in your life. The change you want happens in your now. As you read on, each day you will become more in tune of your habitual ways. And as you complete the daily challenges you can begin to perceive yourself and your life in a different light, you will even begin to notice more balance and a sense of empowerment.

All of these changes will get better each day, and when you are done the 30-day challenge to change you can use this book as your daily guide. Open up to any page and repeat and reinforce the changes you have made to create an even better you and a more joyous life.

Self Love Is the Power That Can Change Your World.

The Power of Self Love

The power of self love can dissolve any negative emotions you have going on within you, moving you in a direction where you can experience joy, happiness, and fulfillment.

The beauty and serenity you experience around you intensifies tenfold with appreciation when you are experiencing the same thing within.

You, however, must begin this process of accepting and approving of who and what you are in the present moment and be ready to happily unfold all the beautiful manifestations that come into your existence.

Live Happily. Love Deeply. Laugh Immensely.

How does one experience this in there life time?

Let's begin by turning on your power and falling in love with yourself. As I often say, falling in love with yourself is the greatest most profound love you will ever experience.

Unfortunately, while love is the core essence of the human race, most people go through life guarded with shields, armours, and walls to protect themselves from pain, hurt, and failures.

Does this resonate with you?

However, the same techniques that protect you, can

also be what's blocking you from experiencing true joy, happiness, and love.

Why would you want to experience anything less than this?

There was a time in my life, when I too believed I would experience greater satisfaction in love and life by protecting myself from pain and hurt. This is a strategy most people use to control what and how they are going to experience and feel.

Ironically, by doing so, it was contrary of what I truly wanted. I was living a mediocre, unsatisfied, and very unhappy life.

Can you relate?

You see, for any change to happen, you must have the willingness to do so. Any kind of joy, happiness, and love you want to attract would mean you must decide to become this person first.

Once you've decided to make yourself a priority, the love within expands, eventually over flowing to all those around you.

Why Is Mindset and Attitude Important?

Having the right mindset and attitude towards how you feel in mind, body, and spirit is the beginning of a very healthy and happy relationship with yourself. After all, you are the only person you can count on one hundred percent to keep you going.

When you are aligned and care about the relationship you have with yourself, my dear friend you are now standing on solid ground.

You see, looking for another person to fulfill you, adore you, reassure you, and love you unconditionally simply means, you have become disconnected with your inner being and are seeking validation externally, through others.

This unrealistic expectation is extremely short lived.

What should you do?

Nourish and take care of you. Make the relationship

with yourself your predominant relationship. You must care about how you feel, learn to reassure yourself, look in the mirror and see your inner beauty and fall in love with yourself from the inside out.

Make the foundation with yourself so strong you will no longer need to look for your rock, your reason for living, or your anchors, because these qualities will already exist within you.

Free others from these titles and conditions, and more importantly, free yourself from depending on others to do what only you are capable of.

Unfold to Possibilities and Trust the Process

For you to create the change you are desiring, your purpose and will to change must become greater. Your thoughts and your body must congruently connect for positive change to occur. When there is a congruency between these two, the intensity of new emotions running through your body can un-program your habitual emotional responses.

You see, your thoughts are the catalytic forces which leads to what your body feels, this force fires up the body to act and create the desire change.

With this new electrifying charge, you can create different exciting experiences, which can awaken different emotions, resulting in growth and breakthroughs, all of which can lead to a more enjoyable, fulfilling, and exciting life.

DAY 1

*Focus on whatever
makes you happy.*

◆ ◆ ◆

Stop waiting for other people to make you happy.

Focus more on one or two things you can do for yourself to spark joy.

Do more of what elevates your happiness, joy, and fulfillment.

DAY 2

Use your memory and your imagination wisely.

◆ ◆ ◆

Today, become aware of how you are using your mind. For example, if you find yourself suddenly drained of your energy, ask yourself what it is you're focussing attention on. Remember energy flows where focus goes.

These two components can either be the foundation for your happiness or your misery.

Remember you can't create a new day with old thoughts. It's a new day for a reason.

DAY 3

Trust the process of allowing.

The greatest thing you can do to attract great manifestations is to ease into the process of "letting it happen."

This takes far less effort and work, as oppose to "making it happen."

Feel the difference already?

Greatness will come to you when you learn to get out of your own way.

Your job is to ask specifically for what you want, then let it be. Trust the universal forces will take care of it. All you must do is be ready and open to receive it when it's delivered.

DAY 4

Listen to your feelings

◆ ◆ ◆

Listen and connect with your inner power of wisdom.

This wisdom is the force you feel leading you on the path of least resistance.

DAY 5

*Do more than belong
in the world*

❖ ❖ ❖

Become an active participant.

Get up and move, do, serve.

It's so easy to sit back and complain about what is not working in your life, relationships, and around the world.

Complaining is a waste of time and energy. If you want to make a difference in your life you have to actively do something that will contribute to change.

For example, if you're in a boring relationship, instead of calling up a friend and complaining how bored you are, set up and plan something to do with your partner. Be aware that when you are feeling bored you are suffering from a lack of growth. You have become complacent, either in your relationship, at work, with your health, finances etc.

Just for today, evaluate an area in your life you are feeling stagnant and become an active participant by doing something that adds value, applicable knowledge, fun, and a shift in your perspective.

DAY 6

Unleash your inner power.

Find out what you are truly capable of.

Sounds EXCITING!

Of course!

Who doesn't like some excitement?

And this is exactly what it can be! Exciting!

Step out of your comfortable self, because you have spent enough time there.

Reach up and go for that bigger and better opportunity because your vibrant passionate self wants to grow, live and experience life on a whole different level.

Here's a suggestion:

Pay attention to your emotional state. This is the best indicator for letting you know it's time for growth.

Get excited for life, an experience only you can create.

DAY 7

Live in your NOW.

◆ ◆ ◆

Every moment is a new starting point.

NOW for happiness.

NOW for doing what you love.

NOW for nourishing your body, mind, and spirit.

Now for surrounding yourself with goodness.

NOW for tapping into your power.

Growth requires a decision to C H A N G E.

How much do you want it?

FRANCA NAVARRA

This is for you to determine.

DAY 8

Live in appreciation.

Living in a state of appreciation simply means, acknowledging where you are right now in life, yet surrendering and trusting the greater forces to lead you towards your ultimate reality.

First thing before you get out of bed, begin with a burst of appreciation by naming anything and everyone you can come up with for five to ten minutes. If you have a hard time, begin with "I appreciate my eyes opening up this morning."

DAY 9

Set one intention as soon as you wake up.

◆ ◆ ◆

The purpose of setting daily intentions is to keep you focused on what matters to you.

What ever the intention, state in terms of what it is you do want, not what you don't. Example...I want to laugh more today vs. I don't want to be so sad.

DAY 1

Care about how you feel.

❖ ❖ ❖

THIS IS PRIORITY.

Get in tune with what you are feeling.

When you care enough about how you feel, self worth kicks in. When self worth kicks in, clarity of what you know you deserve in life powers up.

Celebrate this new found awakening in joy and appreciation.

This profound love begins and ends with you.

...of love is respect, compassion, growth ...ciation, then why settle for anything less ...at you are.

Love yourself first so you know exactly what you deserve.

DAY 11

Stay focus on your vision.

❖ ❖ ❖

Although most people have a clear enough vision, their focus can get shifted by zeroing in on what is not working for them and comparing themselves to others.

STOP!

This is holding you back from experiencing the results you want to achieve.

Why?

When you are functioning in a state of lack and are focused on what others are doing your dominant feeling is not joy, it's envy. This drains your energy, which makes it difficult to become creative and productive.

Your focus must be on your own vision, goals, actions, and outcomes.

Instead of concentrating on what others are working on, create daily healthy habits to keep you inspired and focused on your own dreams.

This is important because it's your daily rituals that get you in the habit of taking consistent daily actions. This is what keeps you going long after the initial excitement of your goal wanes.

Here are the top 4 Principals of Success:

1. Know your outcome.
2. Get in peak state emotionally, mentally and physically.
3. Take action.
4. Be Flexible.

DAY 12

Meditate or sleep

❖ ❖ ❖

Take some time to disconnect with the world, and connect with yours.

When you sleep, mediate or do any activity which quiets the mind you stop all resistance. This gives your mind, body and spirit an opportunity to reconnect, recoup and recharge.

This is the state of being where great achievements are created.

Rehashing and going into the same state of mind

you had before you mediated is a deliberate choice.

DAY 13

Go easy on yourself.

◆ ◆ ◆

You can't un-live what you've lived. So therefore, what you'll be is what you do now.

However, you can use your past experiences as a reference point to create a better life and version of yourself, because what you'll be and experience moving forward depends on what you do now.

DAY 14

Give thanks.

◆ ◆ ◆

There is always something to be thankful for.

Develop a sincere attitude of appreciation. Make a list of all the people, things and places you want to honour, and give a sincere thank you to each one with a warm heart and loving smile.

DAY 15

Make yourself available for only the things that make you feel good.

If it feels right, makes you happy and empowers you, do more of it.

Remember, your thoughts create your emotional state, so let your mind go to where you feel alive.

Cultivate in all things that feel uplifting and delicious in your world.

Bask in what feels good.

DAY 16

Speak in silence.

◆ ◆ ◆

Silence speaks volumes when you want to be heard.

Before responding to someone, take a moment to gather and filter your thoughts. You want your response to come from a place of respect, integrity and love. Most often the best response is the one that is kept quiet.

DAY 17

Tell your loved ones, I love you.

Every breath you take is a second chance to live and appreciate your life.

Tell family, friends, coworkers, acquaintances, and extended family how much you appreciate, love, support, and value them.

It's always so lovely to receive words of endearment, however there is also great joy in giving them to the ones that hold a special place in our heart.

DAY 18

Pamper yourself

◆ ◆ ◆

You first. Take time to take care of your mind, body and spirit. Read, meditate, take a nice warm bath or buy yourself a gift. Nurture and nourish yourself so you can flourish in fulfillment.

This is a must for all you parents out there that believe your children, partner, home, work, friends and extended family must come first before your well being. You must replenish mind, body and spirit in order to give your best to your loved ones happily. Feeling depleted is not a healthy way to serve the ones you love.

Remember yourself throughout the day, so you can be in the best state for those you cherish.

DAY 19

*Trust yourself to
make decisions*

◆ ◆ ◆

Making decisions is inevitable. Everything you have done and continue to do will impact your life. Even when you decide to leave the decision making for someone else, you've decided this too will impact your life.

You know through your own life experiences, decisions have the power to amplify your happiness, fulfillment, joy, or cause misery, tears, and pain.

If you find yourself struggling emotionally and mentally from past decisions, it's time now to apply these four strategies to help you move forward.

1. Change your language. Instead of referring to your past decisions as a mistake, refer to them as life lessons. This sounds and feels a lot better. Does it not?

2. Acknowledge and appreciate your life lessons. Find value in them. You will learn and grow from them every time.

3. Become aware of what you are feeling. Your thoughts and emotions are intertwined.

Replaying your past keeps you stuck on what was and what is. This mindset prevents you from creating what will be.

Find a different focus of attention. Become deliberate about your choice of thoughts. Choose thoughts that create better feeling emotions.

4. Today, trust yourself enough to make a new decision. No matter how big or small, listen to your gut, it will guide you. Most often the first natural response is the correct decision for you. It's when you start to question yourself that you can experience

fear and doubt.

Just know this, whatever you decide, it will be the best decision for you, because the mind goes to what the soul only knows.

Listen for it.

DAY 20

Replace "I will try"
WITH "I will do"

◆ ◆ ◆

TRY leaves room for failure.

Do your thing with a moving forward mindset. This is the mindset needed for all great manifestations to unfold.

DAY 21

Look in the mirror and see your inner beauty and strength.

◆ ◆ ◆

Take five minutes to look at yourself in the mirror and then bring the awareness deeper. Stay there looking at yourself, now go beyond the skin, hair, imperfections. Dive into the eyes of your soul.

What do you see now?

What do you feel?

With a loving gentle voice, tell yourself "I love all of

you." Say it over and over again until you resonate with these words.

Beauty lies within your soul.

Let it radiate vibrantly through you and be felt by those around you.

DAY 22

Wake up and be YOU!

◆ ◆ ◆

Like yourself today, everyone else's likes are extra.

Be funny, joyous, quiet, candid, compassionate... whatever this means to you.

If you are trying to be something for everybody, you are going to end up being nothing for yourself.

So therefore, set the standard of self love high for yourself. Only the people who are qualified will be in your life.

After all, true beauty is being courageous enough to be your authentic self.

From this place of authenticity, everything you do and attract is effortless.

DAY 23

Take a walk in nature.

◆ ◆ ◆

The beauty and serenity you experience around you intensifies tenfold when you are experiencing the same thing within yourself.

Talk about shifting a mood.

A great way to fully embrace the elements of life is to go out and participate with Mother Nature. There is a sense of alignment that takes place within yourself, when you go out and breathe in some fresh air, smell the flowers, and soak up the sun's energy. Connect with yourself as you embrace the elements of life.

DAY 24

Make one smart food choice today.

❖ ❖ ❖

What you choose to eat can determine how you go about your day, the state of mind you'll be in, and the energy you emote.

"Eat to live as oppose to live to eat." Changing this belief can make a huge difference emotionally, mentally, and physically.

When you adapt the belief "eat to live" you will find your perception about food goes deeper than self indulgence and self destruction.

It becomes about nourishing the body, healing, health, self control and most importantly, self love.

All this basically comes down to your decision to do so.

Once your mindset and attitude are aligned, your life will move forward effortless and with pleasure.

You see, most people think change must be done all at once to reap the benefits of transformation.

This is not true.

Small steps and little changes to your day can make a huge difference in your body and how you proceed moving forward.

Start by doing one change a day.

DAY 25

*Forgive yourself for one
thing you did or didn't do.*

❖ ❖ ❖

Whether your decision effected a relationship, your career or finances, you can comfortably shake off any regrets you are holding on to today. This is because these regrettable so-called mistakes are actually life lessons that can repair, rebuild and strengthen the foundation of your life.

Three suggestions to help you move forward.

1. Own what you have done, what you have participated in, and what you have contributed to.

2. Come from a place of appreciation, mentally thank the person and the experience, because it made you wiser and stronger.

3. Focus on what you've learned, and set standards about what you want to live moving forward.

Throughout the course of your life you may need to repeat these steps often. Because you are a full participant of life you must hold yourself accountable for your actions.

DAY 26

*Deliberately surround yourself
only with good vibes.*

◆ ◆ ◆

Like-minded people attract each other, so never become insulted or disappointed when you are not in sync with someone, this simply means your energies are not aligned. One of the biggest reasons for this is that growth has taken place either within you or them.

Two things can happen when this occurs.

1. Remember everyone's light comes on at different times. So eventually your friends or partner will see the change, appreciate it, and will make the change

within themselves as well, allowing you to grow in sync.

Or

2. They are not yet ready for growth and change and may not want to either. This could conjure emotions of unhappiness, loneliness, and resentment which eventually can result in the termination of the friendship or relationship.

Embrace this as it spares you from living with toxicity.

Your inner work now is to deliberately make yourself happy. Find reasons to cultivate in happiness, because vibrating in this state keeps you moving forward to create a joyful and fulfilling life.

DAY 27

*Change one of your
limiting beliefs*

❖ ❖ ❖

Your desired outcomes depend on the beliefs you have about yourself.

If you feel stuck it's because you are stuck. Stuck in the disempowering beliefs that are holding you back from what you desire.

So often, people focus on what they want to achieve while maintaining contrasting beliefs such as "I'm not good enough," "This is impossible," "I'm not smart enough." Can you relate?

These disempowering beliefs create emotions that paralyze you from tapping in to your full potential. This means, any desire, wish, or dream you want to make a reality is forced to remain merely dreams in your head.

Instead, change one belief at a time and replace it with a belief that will empower you emotionally, mentally and physically.

Growth requires you to be willing to create a new way of thinking and speaking about yourself. Without this adjustment you will never tap into what you are fully capable of achieving.

DAY 28

Bring playfulness into everything you do.

◆ ◆ ◆

Find the humour, playfulness, laughter and joy in all that is going on in your external world. Your conditions may not align with what you desire, however, you can make light of any situation by bringing in your playful side and just rolling with it.

DAY 29

Give Back

◆ ◆ ◆

"Let your light shine. Shine within you so that it can shine on someone else. Let your light shine." Oprah Winfrey

In order for you to share your light with someone else, the light must shine bright within you first. You can only give what you are, and when your life is overflowing with abundance, whether it's a smile, compassion, patience, time, or money, you will want to contribute it with the world.

DAY 30

"Celebrate"

❖ ❖ ❖

Celebrate anything great that has happened for you today, no matter how big or small the accomplishment is you must celebrate.

Celebrate with a drink, a nice quiet dinner, by treating yourself to a gift, what ever you must do, do it.

You're training your mind to recognize these great achievements in order for you to create more of them. Whatever you suggest to your mind, your mind starts to look and do more of.

So, let the celebrations begin.

Your inner work can only be determined by you. As you continue to demonstrate this, your love within also expands, gets easier and feels more natural.

Life mirrors back to you the feelings you have inside, so embrace in the knowing that life has your back and it will continue elevating and elating you to your highest goods.

ABOUT THE AUTHOR

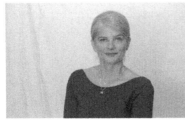

Franca J. Navarra is a certified Master Life Coach, Master Practitioner of Neuro-Linguistic Programming (NLP), International Best Selling Author, Trainer, Motivational Speaker and Yoga Instructor and Reiki Practitioner.

SOURCES AND REFERENCES

❖ ❖ ❖

Dr. Joe Dispenza: Breaking the Habit of Being Yourself, Ester and Jerry Hicks: Ask and it is Given, John C. Maxwell: Put Your Dreams to the Test, Louise Hay: You can Heal Your Life, Oprah Winfrey, Franca J. Navarra: Take Back Your Power training manual

Made in the USA
Monee, IL
15 February 2020